Honey Therapy for Healthy Life

Discover 45 Curable Diseases

with

Pure Natural Honey

By: Ajayi O. Daniel Ph.D.
danielabolaji@gmail.com

HONEY THERAPY FOR HELTHY LIFE

Discover 45 Curable Diseases with Pure Natural Honey

Honey is the natural sweet substance produced by honey bees or a sweet sticky golden-brown fluid produced by bees from the nectar of flowers. This is usually collected in the night.

Honey can be used in cooking, spread on bread, or added to tea. Honey as it is called is the only food source known to contain the twenty-two (22) basic nutrients for balanced nutrition and it is easily assimilated into the blood stream for instant energy production.

Honey contains about 25 essential elements to feed the sensors in the eyes and decrease its tiredness as one age.

The use of honey to enhance proper erection in men is beyond natural medicine as it is proven to contain zinc that is useful for enhancing male sexual organ. Apart from this organic benefit, honey also enhances sound sleep especially when taken with a little volume (8FL OZ) of warm before going to bed. Honey cures dry skin when mix with body cream, supply energy and stamina, aids proper functioning of the liver due to fructose content that secrete glycogen in the liver. It also improves intellect, heals burns and prevents scars and keloid.

More importantly, numerous scientific studies in the global world validate the efficacy of the honey for eye diseases. It is amazing that honey ointments are widely used for various lesions of the cornea. Quite notable numbers of medical practitioners especially in the optical science had also confirmed and authenticated the administering of honey to cure cataract, cornea ulcer, glaucoma and sore eyes. According to Dr. B.G. Gokulan *"honey increases blood circulation in the eyes and tone up the ocular muscles... Honey has excellent healing properties and is highly effective for the treatment of abrasions and ulcer in the cornea"*. By and large honey is referred to as the nerve tonic and could protect the eye of heavy users of computer by countering the harmful effects of radiation. Thus, the unheated raw honey is the only natural honey having enzymes and flavonoids which are potent antioxidant to eliminate free radicals and reverse oxidation of the eye lens protein causing cataract.

INFECTION

1. Athlete's Foot

PRESCRIPTION

Apply pure natural honey on the affected part three times daily until the affected area is healed up.

INFECTION

2. Asthma

PRESCRIPTION

A. Mix one part of castor oil (coconut oil) with five parts of natural honey. Take one spoonful every morning and evening.
B. Mix honey with the clear white liquid of snail. Take two spoonsful three times daily.

INFECTION

    3. Bed-Wetting

PRESCRIPTION

Give the child one spoonful of honey three times daily and two spoonsful at bed.

INFECTION

    4. Boils and Whitlows

PRESCRIPTION

Mix equal parts of honey and flour together. Wrap the affected part with the mixture.

INFECTION

5. Burns

PRESCRIPTION

Smear honey on the affected part at least twice daily.

INFECTION

6. Cold /Catarrh

PRESCRIPTION

Soak slice onion in honey overnight. Take two spoonsful of the mixture three times daily.

INFECTION

7. Cough

PRESCRIPTION

Mix one part of lemon or lime with two spoonsful of honey and lick freely or grind some bitter cola about five (5) pieces and mix the powder with 35cl of natural honey to form a syrup. Three (3) tablespoonful serve three (3) times daily for adult and one (1) tablespoonful serve three (3) times daily for children.

INFECTION

8. Hangover/Drunkenness

PRESCRIPTION

The patient should simply take large amount of honey at thirty (30) minutes interval.

INFECTION

9. Earache

PRESCRIPTION

Apply two drops of honey into the ear and cover with cotton wool. It is best applied at bed time.

Mix small hot water with half tea spoon of salt and honey together apply it with cotton wool before going to bed.

INFECTION

10. Fatigue/Body Weakness

PRESCRIPTION

(a) When you feel tired and weak, make a solution of two spoonful of honey in a glass of lukewarm water and drink. Your energy will be restored.

(b) Take two spoonful of honey every four hours.

INFECTION

11. Gastric Ulcer

PRESCRIPTION

Mix honey and pineapple to make a juice. Take regularly.

12. General Usage

Take honey regularly to strengthen your hear muscle and for brain alertness for quick mastery of things.

INFECTION

13. General Tonic

PRESCRIPTION

Take honey regularly with spur food. Use it for Ogi (akamu, Koko), tea e.t.c.

INFECTION

14. Gum Ache/Pimples

PRESCRIPTION

Boil some honey with onion and lemon juice; add a spoon of salt for 10minutes. Use this solution as a regular mouth wash.

INFECTION

15. Pile (Hemorrhoids)

PRESCRIPTION

Make a charcoal powder of maize cob and mix with honey. Apply as ointment twice daily. It reduces the anal congestion and relieves pain.

INFECTION

16. Hair Loss/Breakage

PRESCRIPTION

Mix equal volume of honey and olive oil. Warm the mixture and massage your hair with it. Rinse the hair with lukewarm water after thirty (30) minutes. Do this forth nightly.

INFECTION

17. Voice Loss/Husky Voice

PRESCRIPTION

(a). Make a mixture of lemon juice with honey. Take two spoonsful at least twice daily.

(b). Mix two spoonsful of honey with one cup of water and boil, breadth over the mixture through the mouth three times daily.

INFECTION

18. Hypertension/High Blood Pressure

PRESCRIPTION

Grind a bulb of garlic and mix with 35cl bottle of honey. Take three spoonsful three times daily.

INFECTION

19. Diabetes

PRESCRIPTION

Make a tea of mistletoe herb. Add two spoonsful of honey with a cup of the tea and drink a cup three times daily for three months.

INFECTION

20. Labor Pains

PRESCRIPTION

Half a cup of pure honey should be taken at the onset of labor.

INFECTION

21. Indigestion

PRESCRIPTION

Take two spoonsful of honey after meal.

INFECTION

22. Insomnia

PRESCRIPTION

Take two spoonsful of honey in a glass of water about one hour before going to bed. Honey relaxes the nerves and ceases tension.

INFECTION

23. Obesity

PRESCRIPTION

Take two spoonful ten minutes before each meal.

INFECTION

24. Libido (Men)

PRESCRIPTION

Make a mixture of two spoonful of honey with four spoonsful of milk and an egg together. Drink the mixture fresh three times daily. It promotes sexual prowess.

INFECTION

25. Malaria

PRESCRIPTION

Mix two spoonsful of honey with two spoonsful of lemon/lime in a glass of water. Drink it after chewing garlic three times daily.

INFECTION

26. Mercy and Favor

Grind Olomisinmisin Leaf well and mix it with honey (1/2 a bottle) Lick it early morning before you talk.

27. Migraine Headache

PRESCRIPTION

Take three spoonsful of honey at the onset of the headache and two spoonsful after thirty (30) minutes.

INFECTION

28. Nasal Bleeding

PRESCRIPTION

Mix one spoonful of honey with one spoonful of onion juice. Breathe it in through the nostrils.

INFECTION

29. Menstrual Pains

PRESCRIPTION

Take two spoonsful of honey every four (4) hours and for three days.

INFECTION

30. General Debility

PRESCRIPTION

Take two or three spoonsful of honey at one-hour intervals.

INFECTION

31. Infertility

PRESCRIPTION

Pure honey taking regularly promotes fertility in women especially when taken along with pollen of bee bread.

INFECTION

32. Irregular or Unstable Menstruation

PRESCRIPTION

Take 2 spoons of honey3 times daily

33. Poison

PRESCRIPTION

Mix equal quantity of honey and palm oil together. This can be taken once as a drink. Honey act as anti-poisonous and emetic in case of poisoning and causes vomiting in which the poison is released.

INFECTION

34. Post Natal Pain

PRESCRIPTION

Take two spoonsful of honey three times daily for three months.

INFECTION

35. Prolonged Menstruation

PRESCRIPTION

Mix honey with half a spoon of cotton pod in warm water. Take this for three days.

INFECTION

36. Rashes (Small Pox, Measles)

PRESCRIPTION

 Mix honey with palm kernel (or palm oil) and smear it on the rashes.

INFECTION

37. Rheumatism

PRESCRIPTION

Grind Bitter leaf and mix it with lime orange water, Ijagain orange water solution. Filter the content and mix with honey (1/2 a coke bottle). Drink half a glass cup and dip clean handkerchief into small solution. Use it to rob/ massage the part of the body that is affected.

38. Sore Throat

PRESCRIPTION

Add honey to a little warmed vinegar and use as a gargle.

INFECTION

39. Tonsillitis (Belu Belu)

PRESCRIPTION

A mixture of honey, grounded cola nut and garlic licked at a regular interval help to reduce the pain of Tonsillitis.

INFECTION

40. Facial Problems (Pimples and others)

PRESCRIPTION

Mix honey with the white part of an egg (albumen) and a few drops of lemon or lime. Use as a face mask and allow to act for thirty (30) minutes before washing the face with lukewarm water.

INFECTION

41. Running Stomach

PRESCRIPTION

Mix honey with orange juice and take two spoonsful three times daily.

INFECTION

42. Constipation

PRESCRIPTION

Mix two spoonsful of honey with a glass cup of milk to which water has been added.

INFECTION

43. Wound and Sores

PRESCRIPTION

Dress the surface of the wound with honey and cover with surgical wool.

INFECTION

44. Tuberculosis

PRESCRIPTION

Ground one bulb of garlic and two bitter cola in 35cl of honey. Take two spoonsful of the solution three times daily.

INFECTION

45. Chapped Hands

PRESCRIPTION

Rub honey on the hands regularly

Reference

Microsoft® Encarta® 2009. © 1993-2008 Microsoft Corporation. All rights reserved.
Preventive and Curative Power in your Daily Diet
The Guardian News Paper

www.ingramcontent.com/pod-product-compliance
Lightning Source LLC
Chambersburg PA
CBHW051933250726
48659CB00002B/989